STRESS AND TENSION

HERBAL REMEDIES

STRESS AND TENSION

MERVYN MITTON

Edited by David Potterton ND, MRN, MNIMH
*Consultant Medical Herbalist and
Registered Naturopath*

foulsham

LONDON · NEW YORK · TORONTO · SYDNEY

foulsham

Yeovil Road, Slough, Berkshire SL1 4JH

ISBN 0-572-01709-X

Printed by St Edmundsbury Press, Bury St Edmunds, Suffolk.
Phototypeset by Typesetting Solutions, Slough, Berks.

Preface

In the early years of this century most medicines were based on herbs. Indeed, many remedies prescribed by doctors had been used with success down the centuries. Even as late as the 1940s about half of all prescriptions still contained herbal ingredients.

During the sixties and seventies, the medical profession began to discard the older, proven methods of treatment in favour of newer chemical-based drugs. Although pharmaceutical research has produced life-saving drugs, there have also been unfortunate results due to the over-reliance on drug therapy for less serious ailments. We now frequently hear reports of side effects — some of them serious — from many of these relatively untested medicines. A number of drugs have had to be withdrawn from the market.

Within the last few years, however, there has been a dramatic resurgence of interest, both from the medical profession and the public, in alternative and complementary forms of treatment, of which herbal medicine remains the most popular.

The aim of this book is to help signpost your way to the many possibilities for safe home treatment with herbs. However, if any doubts about treatment arise it is advisable to seek professional help from a qualified medical herbalist.

The author, Mr Mitton, was a consulting herbalist at Cathay of Bournemouth, a large retail herbal business established by his parents many years ago.

This revised edition of his book gives relevant information and advice to the seeker of good health who wishes to know more about herbal medicine.

Contents

Introduction

Conservative estimates put the number of prescriptions issued each year in the UK for tranquillisers at well over 20,000,000! This is a truly horrendous total, but to understand fully its implications you must also consider that knowledgeable medical opinion and statistics consider the following statements to be substantially accurate.

That one in 50 of the adult population is taking tranquillisers on any day of the year. That approximately one in five women and one in ten men use tranquillisers in the course of a twelve-month period. That a 1982 report by RELEASE estimated that over 100,000 people — mostly women — are addicted to tranquillisers.

The dependence that these drugs create is relieved only by taking further quantities, and therefore it is not unusual to find people who have been taking them for many years. This is despite the fact that many of these drugs lose effectiveness after continued use — some authorities say that this can be as short a time as two months!

The side-effects of the various tranquillising drugs can include anxiety, depression, sexual failure, apprehension, insomnia, and, for some, addiction. Additionally, it can be dangerous to drive or work machinery after taking them, and if alcohol is taken at the same time it can potentiate the side-effects.

When a patient does decide to give up taking them the withdrawal symptoms can include sickness, nausea, headaches, violent shaking, loss of concentration and co-ordination, distorted vision and even suicidal tendencies.

Medical reports show that a common reason for hospital admission is drug overdosage — as high as 15 per cent —

and every year approximately 4,000 people die from taking too many drugs. The extent of the problem can be shown by the example of the City of Portsmouth which in April 1983 collected 3½ tons of unwanted drugs — including nearly a ton of tranquillisers!

The tragedy of all this accumulated misery and self-inflicted illness is that there are alternative forms of treatment available which do not have these side-effects, and herbal treatment is at the forefront of these.

Tension and stress have always been problems, but never more so than with today's pace of life and breakdown of the family unit. With the long history of herbal medicine whereby the possible effects and benefits of a particular remedy have been documented over many years, treatment can be tailored to suit an individual's particular needs and help to reduce tensions and anxieties.

It is important to remember that, used correctly, herbs generally have no side-effects, are not addictive, do not cause depression and do not require ever-increasing dosages to maintain their effect.

The recommendations in this book are based on the known qualities of individual herbs and, in most cases, they can be easily prepared and taken at home. This home treatment approach has a place, since experience has shown that many people prefer to try to control their problems themselves before seeking professional help.

This does not imply that where a serious medical condition exists, it should be treated at home from the advice given in this book. In such a case, you should always contact a medical herbalist or doctor immediately. However, where the pattern of the problem matches examples given, and where the advice is applicable, then herbal treatment could well be the answer.

Chapter 1

Identifying your illness

Most people who suffer from nervous tension and anxiety will have already sought medical advice and have had a correct diagnosis made of their particular problem. However, sometimes complications arise, or the condition is not thought serious enough to worry the doctor, and it is for this reason that a description of the various illnesses and their symptoms are given.

Many readers will be dedicated already to the use of natural medicines, others may have tried alternative treatments without success. The most important thing is to be sure that you have correctly identified your condition before commencing the treatments outlined here as a misdiagnosis could lead to a deterioration in your health. Second, remember that herbal treatment is relatively slow acting and generally relies on a gradual build-up of active principles in the system. This makes it particularly suitable for problems such as nervous tension, since herbs are usually without side-effects, not addictive and are compatible with one another.

ALOPECIA

This is another name for patches of baldness. There can be many contributory causes for this condition, including hereditary factors.

Nervous tension, or severe shock, can also have a serious detrimental effect and often, when tension is present, the hair lacks lustre and becomes dry, brittle and comes out in greater quantities than usual.

Control of nervous tension is of immediate importance together with suitable tonics to restore condition to the hair.

ANOREXIA NERVOSA

This condition usually affects younger women and is triggered by an obsession concerning excessive weight. Symptoms show themselves as a depressed appetite and insomnia.

Herbal nerve treatments can be of assistance, although in some cases psychotherapy or counselling is necessary.

ANXIETY STATES

Generally, these occur when there are constant fears and worries over the most trivial of everyday events.

Herbal treatment can be very helpful.

DEPRESSION

Mental depression is a common illness and can manifest itself in different ways. Severe depression can make the sufferer feel that everyone is unfriendly and lead to immobilisation through fear. This is difficult to treat, and as serious problems, such as suicidal tendencies, are possible, psychotherapy is often necessary.

INSOMNIA

This is an interference with the normal pattern of sleep. Where tensions and anxieties are present they will often be the main contributory factor. A herbal nerve tonic will help to calm the nervous system and a herbal sleeping mixture will induce natural sleep.

MENSTRUAL AND MENOPAUSAL UPSETS

Severe shocks to the nervous system can cause missed menstrual periods. However, the menopausal conditions referred to here are the hot flushes and occasional irritability and depression which can occur.

A combination of St John's Wort and Squaw Weed (one part of each made as an infusion) are traditional specifics for the condition.

NERVOUS DYSPEPSIA

Severe nervous tension can cause an increase in the amount of acid produced in the stomach, and interfere in other ways with the normal digestive processes. This can lead to indigestion, flatulence and general gastric discomfort. Effective herbal treatment will help to control these conditions. A herbal nerve tonic should be taken at the same time.

NERVOUS HEADACHE

This is one of the commonest types of headache and

occurs when an individual becomes tense and worried. The strains of everyday life are often the cause, although women may suffer similar headaches at the menstrual period.

Herbal treatment can be effective when these headaches occur frequently and is generally free of the side-effects of common chemical pain-killers.

NERVOUS TENSION

This is the most commonly encountered nervous problem and one which is likely to affect everyone, with various degrees of severity, at some time. Symptoms can include feelings of inadequacy, sweating and an upset stomach. If allowed to continue for a prolonged period, poor hair and skin, and stomach ulcers can be brought about.

Herbal nerve treatment can be effective without further depressing the nervous system or being addictive.

MIGRAINE

There are many possible factors which trigger migraine attacks. But tension and worry, often allied with fatigue and eye-strain, are major predisposing factors. The condition is often linked too, with certain dairy foods and chocolate.

Our recommendations to patients of the nervous type usually include regular daily intake of a herbal nerve mixture and when an attack starts, this should be augmented for at least a seven-day period by a migraine specific. After a period of time I often find that both the frequency and duration of attacks can be greatly reduced.

TRAVEL SICKNESS

Nervous anticipation can often cause sickness in people undergoing a journey, or the tension, added to the motion of travel, can make the condition more severe. Ginger has always been known for its calming effect on the stomach and the formula for travel sickness given in Chapter 4 has achieved good results.

Chapter 2

Some commonly used drugs

This chapter outlines some of the drugs prescribed by doctors for the treatment of stress and nervous tension together with some of the side effects and adverse reactions associated with them. Some of the drugs listed in the first edition of this book have been withdrawn, or reformulated, or have been replaced by more modern preparations.

The information has not been given to alarm anyone who may be taking any of these drugs, but to make them aware of their possible effects. However, it should be emphasised that people react differently to drugs and that not everyone will, necessarily, suffer side effects.

I believe that many doctors fail to explain fully to their patients the side effects that can be expected from a particular drug, or course of treatment, and that this may cause great distress. This is often due to a failure to communicate since pharmaceutical companies usually advise doctors of the side effects reported during the clinical trials of their medicines.

While there are a number of drugs used for stress and nervous tension which are not listed here, and which are deemed to have fewer or less severe side effects, it should be remembered that all chemical-based drugs are expected to produce side effects.

There is often more than one proprietary brand of a drug, particularly where the patent for the original drug has expired. Brand names are given in brackets.

AMITRIPTYLINE
(Tryptizol)

Indications: Depression in adults.

Possible side effects: May cause dry mouth, constipation, drowsiness, dizziness and weakness. Contraindicated in pregnancy.

CHLORDIAZEPOXIDE
(Librium)

Indications: Short-term therapy for very severe anxiety, with or without insomnia.

Possible side effects: Drowsiness, light-headedness and confusion may occur. Risk of dependency if treatment is continued too long.

CHLORPROMAZINE
(Largactil)

Indications: Acute symptoms of schizophrenia, disturbances requiring sedation, severe emotional disturbances.

Possible side effects: Tremor, muscle spasms, low blood pressure, drowsiness, depression.

DIAZEPAM
(Valium)

Indications: Short-term therapy for severe anxiety with or without insomnia. Nightmares in children.

Possible side effects: Drowsiness, dry mouth, fatigue. Risk of dependency if treatment is continued too long.

GUANETHIDINE
(Ismelin)
Indications: High blood pressure.
Possible side effects: Diarrhoea, dizziness, faintness, slow heart rate, swollen ankles.

HYDROXYZINE
(Atarax)
Indications: Anxiety.
Possible side effects: Drowsiness, dry mouth, headache. Contraindicated in pregnancy.

IMIPRAMINE
(Tofranil)
Indications: Depression, bed-wetting in children.
Possible side effects: Slow-acting drug which may at first increase depression, and cause dry mouth, constipation, blurred vision and fatigue.

IPRINDOLE
(Prondol)
Indications: Depression.
Possible side effects: Similar to imipramine. Contraindicated in people with a history of liver disease.

LABETALOL
(Trandate)

Indications: High blood pressure.

Possible side effects: Care necessary with asthma sufferers.

LORAZEPAM
(Ativan)

Indications: Moderate to severe anxiety.

Possible side effects: Drowsiness, confusion, unsteadiness.

METHYLDOPA
(Aldomet)

Indications: High blood pressure.

Possible side effects: Headache, depression, drowsiness, nasal congestion, dry mouth.

MIANSERIN
(Bolvidon)
(Norval)

Indications: Depression.

Possible side effects: Drowsiness, blood disorders.

NITRAZEPAM
(Mogadon)

Indications: Short-term therapy for severe insomnia.

Possible side effects: Drowsiness, unsteadiness. Risk of dependency if treatment is continued too long.

OXAZEPAM
Indications: Anxiety.
Possible side effects: Drowsiness, confusion, unsteadiness, dizziness.

OXYPERTINE
(Integrin)
Indications: Anxiety, delirium, neuroses and psychoses.
Possible side effects: Affects judgement, and may cause drowsiness or agitation, bouts of low blood pressure, dizziness and vomiting.

PERPHENAZINE
(Fentazin)
Indications: Anxiety and tension, schizophrenia.
Possible side effects: Muscle spasms, stomach upsets, dry mouth, blurred vision, agitation.

PHENELZINE
(Nardil)
Indications: Depression and phobias.
Possible side effects: Headache, drowsiness, fatigue, constipation, restlessness. May increase action of other drugs and interact with foods, particularly cheese, meat and yeast extracts.

PROCHLORPERAZINE
(Stemetil)

Indications: Minor emotional and mental upsets, schizophrenia. Also indicated for nausea and vomiting.

Possible side effects: Muscle spasms, tremors, drowsiness.

RESERPINE

Indications: High blood pressure.

Possible side effects: Depression, lethargy, stomach ulcers, diarrhoea, nasal congestion.

Chapter 3

Some problems which trouble sufferers

People who suffer nervous complaints do not need to be told of the many side-effects which can occur as a result of treatment for the original nerve trouble. Even so, I often find that patients who come for consultations have not associated their specific health problems with the original nervous condition. This means, of course, that when they are seeking treatment — either from a chemist or consulting their doctors — they are dealing with each illness as a separate issue, instead of looking for balanced overall treatment.

I have already mentioned that vast numbers of prescriptions are issued for tranquillising tablets, all of which can produce disturbing side-effects. These potential side-effects must be taken into account, since their effect is often to make the patient think they have a separate illness and, in turn, look for treatment for this. The result can be even more unnecessary drugs being introduced into the system.

Herbal treatment is generally without side-effects and after so many years of use, those that are present are fully understood. For this reason, herbal treatment is particularly suitable for nervous based problems, since it is not addictive, does not add to problems already present by causing depression, does not require continually increasing dosages to maintain benefits and is generally compatible with other herbal medicines and, indeed, with most chemical medicines which may also have to be taken.

There are three main ways in which nervous tension and anxieties can lead to additional illness; obviously, there can be others, but for someone considering home treatment, these are the three of greatest importance.

HAIR

It is well known that a severe shock can lead to hair loss, or even a loss of colour to white or grey virtually overnight. Unfortunately, not many sufferers of severe nervous tension realise that it can also affect the general condition of their hair. There can be a marked loss of condition when a person is under tension, usually the hair losing its gloss and becoming dry and brittle. Accelerated hair loss is often noticed when the hair is combed or brushed and baldness can quickly become apparent.

SKIN AILMENTS

Psoriasis and eczema can be directly linked with tension and, indeed, its onset can often be traced back to a severe emotional shock, such as a death in the family, or perhaps a divorce. Psoriasis is particularly difficult to treat. It often appears to clear spontaneously, but at times of emotional disturbance, perhaps even years later, may recur.

STOMACH ULCERS

When extremes of tension are experienced, particularly over a long period of time, the digestive processes of the stomach are disturbed. There are always amounts of acid present in the stomach which are necessary to help process food. But at times of tension, additional acid can be created which can attack the linings of the stomach and eventually cause ulcers to develop.

TREATMENTS

Specific treatments are recommended for the above health problems in both this book and in other volumes in this series. However, it is stressed that to treat any of the above three without attention to the nervous problem which caused them in the first place is unlikely to be effective. Herbal medicine is considered to be a complete approach to treatment for not only the effect but also the original cause, and, for this reason, it is often successful where other medicines fail.

Chapter 4

Herbal treatments and medication

The preparations in this chapter can be made at home following the given instructions and using quantities shown as percentages of the overall herb weight.

Ingredients should be available from herbal suppliers and many health food shops. If any difficulty is experienced consult the list of addresses at the back of the book.

INFORMATION ON THE PREPARATION OF HERBS

DECOCTIONS

The herbs, usually the roots and bark, are cut, ground up or bruised and covered with cold fresh water. This mixture is then boiled for up to half an hour, allowed to cool and then strained through a fine mesh. Allow 28 grams of the herbs to 568 ml of water (1 oz to 1 pint). This method is used when the herb is unsuitable to make as an infusion. The usual dose is one small wineglassful three times daily.

INFUSIONS

Teas or tisanes are made by the process of infusion. Prepare the herbs to be used and quickly pour boiling water on them. Allow the mixture to stand for about half an hour, stirring frequently and when ready strain off the liquid. Allow 28 grams to 568 ml of water (1 oz to 1 pint). The usual dose is approximately one small teacup or wineglassful three times daily, usually one after each main meal.

SOLID EXTRACTS
Start with a strong infusion of the herbs required and evaporate over low heat until a heavy consistency is obtained.

TINCTURES
This process is used for herbs and drugs which become useless when heated, or for those herbs which are not amenable to treatment by water. Tinctures are made commercially with pure alcohol. Use 28 to 56 grams to 568 ml (1 to 2 oz to 1 pint). The dose varies according to strength of main ingredient. For home use tinctures can be made with brandy, but this is rather an expensive process.

SOME SIMPLE FORMULAE TO MAKE AT HOME

A GOOD GENERAL HERB MIXTURE FOR NERVOUS TENSION

Motherwort	1 part
Hops	1 part
Vervain	1 part
Lime Flowers	1 part
Scullcap	1 part

Make up as an infusion.

A HERB MIXTURE FOR NERVOUS HEADACHES

Betony	1 part
Scullcap	1 part
Valerian	1 part

Make up as an infusion.

A HERB MIXTURE FOR MIGRAINOUS HEADACHES

Rosemary	1 part
Valerian	1 part
Lavender Flowers	½ part
Lady's Slipper	1 part

Make up as an infusion.

A HERB MIXTURE FOR DEPRESSION

Oats (Avena)	1 part
Damiana (Turnera)	1 part
Kola	1 part
Rosemary	1 part

Make up as an infusion.

A HERB MIXTURE FOR NERVOUS EXCITABILITY AND ANXIETY

Cowslip Flowers (Primula)	1 part
Valerian	1 part
Lady's Slipper	1 part
Scullcap	1 part
Hops	1 part

Make up as an infusion.

A HERB MIXTURE FOR INSOMNIA

Hops	1 part
Pulsatilla	1 part
Cowslip Flowers (Primula)	1 part
Vervain	1 part

Make up as an infusion.

A HERB MIXTURE FOR THE MENOPAUSE

St John's Wort	1 part
Squaw Weed	1 part
Pulsatilla	1 part

Make up as an infusion.

A HERB MIXTURE FOR TRAVEL SICKNESS

German Chamomile	1 part
Ginger	1 part

Make up as an infusion.

A HERB MIXTURE FOR NERVOUS DYSPEPSIA

Belgian Chamomile	1 part
Hops	1 part
Marshmallow	1 part
Lemon Balm	1 part
Meadowsweet	1 part

Make up as an infusion.

A HERB MIXTURE FOR PSORIASIS

Mountain Grape	1 part
Burdock Root	1 part
Yellow Dock Root	1 part
Red Clover Flowers	1 part
Sarsaparilla	1 part

Make up as an infusion.

Chapter 5

Some recommended herbs

This section of the book lists in alphabetical order herbs which can be used in the treatment of the conditions mentioned earlier, together with other herbs of a generally beneficial nature.

A list of herbal suppliers is given at the end of the section. A few herbs may be available only on prescription from a medical herbalist.

Mitton's Practical Modern Herbal, published by Foulsham, is recommended for a more complete list of medical herbs and their uses, together with much useful information.

Acacia Gum
ACACIA SENEGAL

Also known as	Gum Arabic.
Found wild	North Africa.
Appearance	Round tears obtained from spring shrub. Cuts are made in the bark and the gum exudes and coagulates.
Part used	Coagulated gum.
Therapeutic uses	An excellent demulcent, often used to relieve catarrh and chest complaints.
Prepared as	Mucilage by combining with hot water.

29

Adder's Tongue, American
ERYTHRONIUM AMERICANUM

Also known as	Snake's Tongue.
Found wild	North America.
Appearance	Small bulbous plant with only two leaves; bright yellow lily-like flowers.
Part used	Leaves.
Therapeutic uses	Generally as a poultice for ulcers and skin troubles.
Prepared as	Poultice.

Agar-Agar
GELIDIUM AMANSII

Also known as	Japanese Isinglass.
Found wild	Japan.
Appearance	Prepared from a compound of several different seaweeds into thin strips of about 30 cm long from dried jelly.
Part used	Translucent strips.
Therapeutic uses	Excellent for relief of stubborn constipation.
Prepared as	Powder.

Agrimony
AGRIMONIA EUPATORIA

Also known as	Sticklewort.

Found wild	Throughout northern Europe.
Appearance	A strong-growing herb with green-grey leaves covered with soft hairs. Flowers are small and yellow on long slender spikes.
Part used	Herb.
Therapeutic uses	Dried leaves when infused make an astringent useful for diarrhoea; also as a tonic and diuretic.
Prepared as	Infusion.

Alder, English
ALNUS GLUTINOSA

Found wild	England, Europe and North Africa.
Appearance	A small tree of distinctive appearance.
Parts used	Bark and leaves.
Therapeutic uses	The bark is used as a cathartic and the leaves to treat inflammation.
Prepared as	Decoction and poultice.

Alstonia Bark
ALSTONIA CONSTRICTA

Also known as	Fever Bark and Australia Quinine.
Found wild	Australia.
Appearance	Thick chocolate-coloured spongy bark from a moderate-sized tree.

Part used	Bark.
Therapeutic uses	To prevent recurring bouts of malaria and for quick and effective relief of most forms of rheumatism.
Prepared as	Powder or decoction.

Amaranth
AMARANTHUS HYPOCHONDRIACUS

Also known as	Love Lies Bleeding.
Found wild	UK and Europe.
Appearance	A common garden plant with crimson flowers similar to a coxscomb.
Part used	Herb.
Therapeutic uses	Treatment of diarrhoea and menorrhagia. As an astringent. Helpful in all cases of looseness of the bowel.
Prepared as	Decoction.

Ammoniacum
DOREMA AMMONIACUM

Also known as	Gum Ammoniacum.
Found wild	Turkey and Iran.
Appearance	Small rounded lumps, pale yellow in colour, browning with age.
Part used	Gum resin.

| **Therapeutic uses** | For respiratory troubles. Used in particular for the relief of catarrh, asthma and bronchitis. |
| **Prepared as** | Powder. |

Angelica
ANGELICA ARCHANGELICA

Found wild	Europe and Asia.
Appearance	Plant growing from one and a half to two metres high.
Parts used	Root, seeds and herb.
Therapeutic uses	For rheumatic diseases, catarrh and asthma. A stimulant and diaphoretic.
Prepared as	Infusion or decoction.

Aniseed
PIMPINELLA ANISUM

Found wild	Europe, North Africa.
Appearance	An umbelliferous plant with serrated leaves. Small brownish-grey seeds.
Part used	Fruit.
Therapeutic uses	A pectoral. used for cough medicines and elixirs.
Prepared as	Powder or decoction.

Angostura
GALIPEA OFFICINALIS

Found wild	South America.
Appearance	A diminutive hardy tree. Bark when stripped has a tobacco-like odour.
Part used	Bark.
Therapeutic uses	As a tonic and a cathartic.
Prepared as	Decoction.

Aniseed
PIMPINELLA ANISUM

Found wild	Europe and North Africa.
Appearance	An umbelliferous plant with serrated leaves and small brownish grey seeds.
Part used	Fruit.
Therapeutic uses	A pectoral, used for cough medicines and elixirs.
Prepared as	Decoction.

Arrach
CHENOPODIUM OLIDUM

Also known as	Goat's Arrach.
Found wild	Throughout Europe.
Appearance	A small inconspicuous herb with an unpleasant odour.

Part used	Herb.
Therapeutic uses	As an emmenagogue to bring on menstruation. Also an effective nervine.
Prepared as	Infusion.

Asafoetida
FERULA FOETIDA

Found wild	Iran and the Himalayas.
Appearance	Grown in clumps to 2m/7ft high. Odour like Garlic.
Part used	Gum resin.
Therapeutic uses	A stimulant and antispasmodic, often used to relieve croup and colic.
Prepared as	Powder or tincture. Pills are better.

Avens
GEUM URBANUM

Also known as	Colewort.
Found wild	Throughout Europe.
Appearance	Low-growing herb with yellow flowers.
Parts used	Herb and root.
Therapeutic uses	To stay bleeding and as a reliable tonic for women. Also used for treating leucorrhea.
Prepared as	Decoction.

Part used	Leaves.
Therapeutic uses	Regarded as one of the best remedies for liver diseases. It is also antibilious, anthelmintic and a tonic.
Prepared as	Infusion.

Bayberry
MYRICA CERIFERA

Also known as	Waxberry, Candleberry.
Found wild	Europe and North America.
Appearance	A medium-growing shrub with a profusion of large white berries.
Part used	Bark.
Therapeutic uses	A strong stimulant. A warming and effective deobstruent and cleanser. Also as a poultice for ulcers.
Prepared as	Infusion and poultice.

Bearsfoot, American
POLYMNIA UVEDALIA

Also known as	Yellow Leaf Cup.
Found wild	North America.
Appearance	A tall branching plant found in loamy soil.
Part used	Root.
Therapeutic uses	For quick pain relief, as a gentle laxative for the aged and as a stimulant.
Prepared as	Decoction.

Betony
BETONICA OFFICINALIS

Also known as	Wood Betony.
Found wild	UK and Europe.
Appearance	Plant growing to 60 cm. Long leaves with spiky flowers.
Part used	Herb.
Therapeutic uses	As a sedative, astringent and alterative. Of value for treatment of headaches and anxiety.
Prepared as	Infusion.

Birch, European
BETULA ALBA

Found wild	Europe.
Appearance	A strikingly handsome tree common on gravel soils. Distinctive black and white bark.
Parts used	Bark and leaves.
Therapeutic uses	Birch tar oil makes a soothing oitment for skin disorders. The bark, as an infusion, is good for kidney stones.
Prepared as	Infusion and oil.

Bistort
POLYGONUM BISTORTA

Also known as	Adderwort.
Found wild	Europe and northern Britain.

Appearance	A tall, branching plant found in rich loamy soil.
Part used	Root.
Therapeutic uses	Used for pain relief and as a gentle laxative. Also used in ointments for scalp conditions.
Prepared as	Decoction.

Beth Root
TRILLIUM ERECTUM

Also known as	Birthroot.
Found wild	Northern USA.
Appearance	Low-growing herb.
Part used	Rhizome.
Therapeutic uses	A tonic and stimulant. Will help to allay excessive menstruation. Used externally for ulcers.
Prepared as	Infusion, poultice and ointment.

Birch (European)
BETULA ALBA

Found wild	Europe.
Appearance	A strikingly handsome tree common on gravel soils, with distinctive black and white bark.
Parts used	Bark and leaves.
Therapeutic uses	Birch tar oil makes a soothing oitment for skin disorders. The bark, as an infusion, is good for kidney stones.
Prepared as	Infusion or oil.

Bistort
POLYGONUM BISTORTA

Also known as	Adderwort.
Found wild	Europe and Northern Great Britain.
Appearance	Low-growing herb chiefly found in ditches and damp places.
Part used	Root.
Therapeutic uses	A useful treatment for incontinence. Also used as a gargle for sore throats.
Prepared as	Decoction.

Bitter Root
APOCYNUM ANDROSAEMIFOLIUM

Also known as	Dogsband, Fly Trap.
Found wild	North America.
Appearance	A woody herb with acuminate leaves.
Part used	Root.
Therapeutic uses	A cathartic and heart tonic. Also a powerful emetic and diuretic.
Prepared as	Decoction.

Black Root
LEPTANDRA VIRGINICA

Also known as	Culver's Root.

Borage
BORAGO OFFICINALIS

Also known as	Burrage.
Found wild	Throughout Europe.
Appearance	Bold, erect herb of strong growth. Small blue flowers.
Part used	Leaves.
Therapeutic uses	As a tonic and stimulant. Also as a remedy for migraine and headaches.
Prepared as	Decoction or powder.

Boxwood, American
CORNUS FLORIDA

Also known as	Dogwood and Cornel.
Found wild	United States.
Appearance	Small tree with rough bark and a profusion of pink spring flowers.
Parts used	Root and bark.
Therapeutic uses	As a tonic and stimulant. Also as a remedy for migraine and headaches.
Prepared as	Decoction or powder.

Broom
CYTISUS SCOPARIUS

Also known as	Irish Broom.
Found wild	Throughout Europe.

Appearance	A small graceful arching shrub with profuse floral display.
Part used	Top of each sprig.
Therapeutic uses	As a diuretic and cathartic. Also used for the relief of liver troubles and fluid retention. May affect blood pressure.
Prepared as	Infusion.

Buchu
BAROSMA BETULINA

Also known as	Bucco.
Found wild	Western coast of South Africa.
Appearance	Small procumbent herb growing in dry places.
Part used	Leaves.
Therapeutic uses	Urinary and bladder troubles. Also a diaphoretic and stimulant.
Prepared as	Infusion or decoction.

Bugle
AJUGA REPTANS

Also known as	Sicklewort.
Found wild	European woodlands.
Appearance	Diminutive herb with distinctive square stems and blue flower.
Part used	Herb.
Therapeutic uses	An astringent.
Prepared as	Infusion.

Boxwood (American)
CORNUS FLORIDA

Also known as	Dogwood, Cornel.
Found wild	United States.
Appearance	Small tree with rough bark and a profusion of pink spring flowers.
Parts used	Root and bark.
Therapeutic uses	As a tonic or stimulant and as a remedy for migraine and headaches.
Prepared as	Decoction or powder.

Broom
CYTISUS SCOPARIUS

Also known as	Irish Broom.
Found wild	Throughout Europe.
Appearance	A small, graceful, arching shrub with profuse floral display.
Part used	Top of each sprig.
Therapeutic uses	A diuretic and cathartic. Also used for relief of liver troubles and fluid retention. May affect blood pressure.
Prepared as	Infusion.

Buchu
BAROSMA BETULINA

Also known as	Bucco.
Found wild	Western coast of South Africa.

Appearance	Small procumbent herb growing in dry places.
Part used	Leaves.
Therapeutic uses	For urinary and bladder troubles. Also a diaphoretic and stimulant.
Prepared as	Infusion or decoction.

Bugle
AJUGA REPTANS

Also known as	Sicklewort.
Found wild	European woodlands.
Appearance	Diminutive herb with distinctive square stems and blue flowers.
Part used	Herb.
Therapeutic uses	An astringent.
Prepared as	Infusion.

Bugloss
ECHIUM VULGARE

Also known as	Viper's Bugloss.
Found wild	Europe.
Appearance	A sturdy herb with blue flowers.
Part used	Herb.
Therapeutic uses	An expectorant and demulcent. Excellent for gentle bowel action. Also to clear phlegm from bronchial tubes.
Prepared as	Infusion.

Caroba
JACARANDA PROCERA

Also known as	Carob Tree.
Found wild	South Africa and South America.
Appearance	A handsome tree with lanceolate leaves.
Part used	Leaves.
Therapeutic uses	As a diaphoretic and diuretic. Also a sedative.
Prepared as	Infusion.

Cascarilla
CROTON ELEUTERIA

Also known as	Sweet Wood Bark.
Found wild	The Bahamas and West Indies.
Appearance	A diminutive tree.
Part used	Bark.
Therapeutic uses	A tonic stimulant.
Prepared as	Decoction.

Catnip
NEPETA CATARIA

Also known as	Catmint.
Found wild	Britain.
Appearance	A procumbent grey plant.
Part used	Herb.

| **Therapeutic uses** | Carminative and diaphoretic and has tonic properties. Also used for the relief of piles. |
| **Prepared as** | Infusion. |

Cayenne, Hungarian
CAPSICUM TETRAGONUM

Also known as	Paprika.
Found wild	Hungary, also cultivated elsewhere.
Appearance	A strong-growing herb with large green fruits.
Part used	Fruit.
Therapeutic uses	Rich source of vitamin C.
Prepared as	Powder. Small doses.

Centaury
ERYTHRAEA CENTAURIUM

Also known as	Feverwort.
Found wild	UK and Europe.
Appearance	Small pink-flowered herb.
Part used	Leaves.
Therapeutic uses	Stomachic, aromatic, bitter. For stomach upsets and anorexia nervosa.
Prepared as	Infusion.

Cascarilla
CROTON ELEUTERIA

Also known as	Sweet Wood Bark.
Found wild	West Indies (Bahamas only).
Appearance	A diminutive tree.
Part used	Bark.
Therapeutic uses	A tonic stimulant.
Prepared as	Decoction.

Catnip
NEPETA CATARIA

Also known as	Catmint.
Found wild	Great Britain.
Appearance	A procumbent grey plant.
Part used	Herb.
Therapeutic uses	A carminative and diaphoretic, with tonic properties. Also used for the relief of piles.
Prepared as	Infusion.

Cayenne, Hungarian
CAPSICUM TETRAGONUM

Also known as	Paprika.
Found wild	Hungary. Also cultivated.
Appearance	A strong-growing herb with large green fruits.
Part used	Fruit.
Therapeutic uses	Rich source of vitamin C.
Prepared as	Powder. Small doses.

Chamomile (Belgian)
ANTHEMIS NOBILIS

Found wild	Belgium and France. Widely cultivated.
Appearance	Herb with double flowers.
Part used	Flower.
Therapeutic uses	Widely used for women suffering from nervous upsets and as a tonic, stomachic and antispasmodic.
Prepared as	Infusion.

Chamomile (German)
MATRICARIA CHAMOMILLA

Found wild	Europe.
Appearance	Herb with small cushion-like flowers in profusion.
Part used	Flowers.
Therapeutic uses	Excellent nerve sedative, carminative and tonic. Also used as a poultice for leg ulcers.
Prepared as	Infusion or poultice.

Chickweed
STELLARIA MEDIA

Also known as	Starweed.
Found wild	Great Britain.

Cloves
EUGENIA CARYOPHYLLUS

Found wild	Zanzibar, Madagascar and the East Indies.
Appearance	Beautiful evergreen tree of majestic appearance.
Part used	Flower, buds and oil.
Therapeutic uses	A stimulant and carminative usually compounded with other remedies.
Prepared as	Oil and spice.

Clubmoss
LYCOPODIUM CLAVATUM

Found wild	Northern hemisphere.
Appearance	Low spreading greyish-green plant usually found near water.
Part used	Herb.
Therapeutic uses	Treatment of cystitis, kidney complaints and urinary disorders. Also a sedative and for stomach disorders.
Prepared as	Infusion.

Cohosh, Blue
CAULOPHYLLUM THALICTROIDES

Also known as	Blueberry Root.
Found wild	United States and Canada.

Appearance	A gnarled, crowded shrub.
Part used	Rhizome.
Therapeutic uses	As a diuretic and emmenagogue, also as a vermifuge to expel worms. Aids rheumatic sufferers and menstrual problems.
Prepared as	Decoction.

Comfrey
SYMPHYTUM OFFICINALE

Also known as	Knitbone and Slippery Root.
Found wild	Throughout UK and Europe.
Appearance	Fleshy-leaved plant about one metre high.
Parts used	Leaves and root.
Therapeutic uses	Helpful for treatment of internal ulcers. For rheumatic pains and for arthritis and a poultice for treatment of bruises and sprains.
Prepared as	Decoction and poultice.

Condurango
MARSDENIA CONDURANGO

Found wild	South America.
Appearance	Nondescript climbing vine found in heavily forested areas.
Part used	Bark.
Therapeutic uses	An alterative and stomachic. Helpful for treating duodenal ulcers.
Prepared as	Decoction or powder.

49

Therapeutic uses	As a diuretic and emmenagogue. Also as a vermifuge. Aids rheumatic sufferers. For women suffering from amenorrhea and dysmenorrhea.
Prepared as	Decoction.

Comfrey
SYMPHYTUM OFFICINALE

Also known as	Knitbone, Slippery Root.
Found wild	Throughout UK and Europe.
Appearance	Fleshy-leaved plant which can grow to approximately 91 cm/ three feet.
Parts used	Leaves and root.
Therapeutic uses	Helpful for treatment of internal and external ulcers. For rheumatic pains, arthritis and as a poultice for the treatment of bruises and sprains.
Prepared as	Decoction, poultice and ointment.

Condurango
MARSDENIA CONDURANGO

Found wild	South America.
Appearance	Nondescript climbing vine found in heavily forested areas.
Part used	Bark.
Therapeutic uses	As alterative and stomachic. Helpful for treating duodenal ulcers.
Prepared as	Decoction.

Cotton Root
GOSSYPIUM HERBACEUM

Found wild	Mediterranean islands and United States.
Appearance	Twists of bark.
Part used	Bark of root.
Therapeutic uses	Treatment of women's disorders including amenorrhea or dysmenorrhea.
Prepared as	Infusion.

Cramp Bark
VIBURNUM OPULUS

Also known as	Snow-ball Tree, Guelder Rose.
Found wild	Europe and America.
Appearance	Strong-growing bush with white ball-shaped flowers.
Part used	Bark.
Therapeutic uses	As a nervine for treatment of spasms and convulsions. Antispasmodic. Regarded as a safe children's medication.
Prepared as	Decoction.

Cranesbill (American)
GERANIUM MACULATUM

Also known as	Wild Geranium or Storksbill.
Found wild	United States.
Appearance	Shrubby small herb with blue flowers.

Damiana
TURNERA DIFFUSA

Found wild	Southern USA and Mexico.
Appearance	Medium-sized shrub.
Parts used	Leaves and stem.
Therapeutic uses	Aphrodisiac. Tonic. Anti-depressant.
Prepared as	Infusion.

Dandelion
TARAXACUM OFFICINALE

Found wild	Most temperate climates.
Appearance	Common herb with long root, toothed leaves and bright yellow flowers.
Parts used	Leaves and root.
Therapeutic uses	As a tonic and diuretic and for liver and kidney ills. Roots frequently used for coffee as it contains no caffeine.
Prepared as	Infusion or decoction.

Dodder
CUSCUTA EPITHYMUM

Found wild	Throughout the world.
Appearance	A climbing parasite of the convolvulus family.
Part used	Herb.

| **Therapeutic uses** | As a mild laxative and hepatic and for the treatment of bladder and liver troubles. |
| **Prepared as** | Infusion. |

Dog Rose
ROSA CANINA

Also known as	Wild Briar.
Found wild	Europe and the Middle East.
Appearance	The wild rambling rose.
Part used	Fruit.
Therapeutic uses	The fruit yields ascorbic acid (vitamin C) of particular value when given to young children.
Prepared as	Syrup.

Echinacea
ECHINACEA ANGUSTIFOLIA

Also known as	Coneflower.
Found wild	United States.
Appearance	Herb of medium height.
Part used	Rhizome.
Therapeutic uses	Antiseptic and alterative and to help purify the blood. Used for boils and carbuncles.
Prepared as	Decoction.

Therapeutic uses	For colds and influenza and as an alterative. It is a safe soporific and induces healthy sleep.
Prepared as	Infusion.

Evening Primrose
OENOTHERA BIENNIS

Also known as	Tree Primrose.
Found wild	European gardens.
Appearance	Small herb with a delightful display of yellow flowers.
Parts used	Leaves, bark and oil.
Therapeutic uses	As a sedative and astringent. Also used for menstrual disorders and skin diseases.
Prepared as	Decoction, oil (available in capsules).

Fenugreek
TRIGONELLA FOENUM-GRAECUM

Found wild	Mediterranean area, North Africa and India.
Appearance	Slender-stemmed plant.
Part used	Herb.
Therapeutic uses	As an emolient, a laxative and expectorant. Can be applied externally to assist gout, ulcers, wounds and boils.
Prepared as	Decoction and poultice.

Feverfew
CRYSANTHEMUM PARTHENIUM

Also known as	Featherfew.
Found wild	Throughout Europe.
Appearance	A small, grey herb with hairy stems.
Part used	Herb.
Therapeutic uses	As an aperient. Also used by women to bring on the menses. Now recognised as an aid to migraine.
Prepared as	Infusion.

Figwort
SCROPHULARIA NODOSA

Also known as	Throatwort.
Found wild	Throughout Europe.
Appearance	Medium-sized tree of rampant growth.
Part used	Herb.
Therapeutic uses	Aperient. Also an emollient and demulcent, and as a poultice for ulcers. Helpful for chronic skin complaints.
Prepared as	Infusion or poultice.

Fringetree
CHIONANTHUS VIRGINICA

Found wild	Southern United States.

Appearance	Medium-sized tree of rampant growth.
Part used	Herb.
Therapeutic uses	Aperient, also an emollient and demulcent and as a poultice for ulcers. Helpful for chronic skin complaints.
Prepared as	Infusion and poultice.

Fringetree
CHIONANTHUS VIRGINICA

Found wild	Southern United States.
Appearance	A small tree with inconspicuous white flowers. It has a very bitter taste.
Part used	The bark of the root.
Therapeutic uses	Tonic, alterative and diuretic. Also for treatment of liver disorders, gallstones and jaundice.
Prepared as	Decoction.

Garlic
ALLIUM SATIVUM

Where found	Universally cultivated.
Appearance	Similar to a shallot.
Part used	Bulb.
Therapeutic uses	For treatment of dyspepsia and flatulence, also as a stimulant. Reduces cholesterol in the blood.
Prepared as	Juice and tincture.

Gentian
GENTIANA LUTEA

Found wild	Alpine meadows.
Appearance	A plant with oblong pale green leaves and large, yellow scented flowers.
Part used	Root.
Therapeutic use	Tonic.
Prepared as	Decoction or powder.

Germander
TEUCRIUM CHAMAEDRYS

Also known as	Wall Germander.
Found wild	UK and Europe.
Appearance	Stemmed plant growing to about half a metre.
Part used	Herb.
Therapeutic uses	A helpful plant for the treatment of rheumatoid arthritis and gout. Has anti-inflammatory properties.
Prepared as	Decoction.

Ginger
ZINGIBER OFFICINALE

Found wild	West Indies and China.
Appearance	About one metre high with glossy aromatic leaves.
Part used	Rhizome.

Therapeutic uses	Has stimulative and carminative properties. Can be used as an expectorant and an aid to digestion.
Prepared as	Powder or decoction.

Golden Seal
HYDRASTIS CANADENSIS

Also known as	Yellow Root.
Where found	Cultivated in North America.
Appearance	Tall-growing herb with disagreeable odour.
Part used	Rhizome.
Therapeutic uses	For skin and gastric disorders and as a soothing laxative and tonic.
Prepared as	Decoction or powder.

Guarana
PAULLINIA CUPANA

Also known as	Brazilian Cocoa.
Found wild	Brazil.
Appearance	A tall arching shrub.
Part used	Seeds.
Therapeutic uses	As a stimulant and for relief of headaches and migraine. Also used by women to bring on the menses and can be effective in the treatment of arthritis.
Prepared as	Decoction.

Hawthorn
CRATAEGUS OXYCANTHA

Also known as	May Tree.
Found wild	Throughout Britain.
Appearance	A common small tree.
Part used	Fruit.
Therapeutic use	As an aid for heart conditions.
Prepared as	Decoction.

Heartsease
VIOLA TRICOLOR

Also known as	Wild Pansy.
Found wild	UK.
Appearance	Similar to garden pansy.
Parts used	Stem and leaves.
Therapeutic uses	A diuretic and anti-rheumatic. Eczema and skin eruptions can be treated with it by external application.
Prepared as	Infusion.

Holy Thistle
CARBENIA BENEDICTA

Also known as	Blessed Thistle.
Found wild	Southern Europe.
Appearance	Typical thistle.

Therapeutic uses	A safe emmenagogue and diaphonetic. Helpful externally for ulcers.
Prepared as	Infusion.

Hops
HUMULUS LUPULUS

Found wild	Europe and cultivated in most parts of the world.
Appearance	A climbing vine.
Part used	Strobiles.
Therapeutic uses	An anodyne for the relief of pain. A tonic, an aid for stomach disorders and to promote sleep.
Prepared as	Infusion.

Horseradish
COCHLEARIA ARMORACIA

Found wild	Europe.
Appearance	A herb growing to one metre with a pungent odour.
Part used	Root.
Therapeutic uses	Relieves flatulence and indigestion. Promotes perspiration and is a diuretic.
Prepared as	Infusion.

Horsetail
EQUISETUM ARVENSE

Also known as	Scouring Rushes.

Found wild	Britain.
Appearance	A tall bold herb with cane-like appearance.
Part used	Herb.
Therapeutic uses	A powerful astringent and also a diuretic. Excellent for kidney troubles.
Prepared as	Decoction.

Houndstongue
CYNOGLOSSUM OFFICINALE

Found wild	Britain.
Appearance	A medium-sized herb with long, strap-like leaves.
Part used	Herb.
Therapeutic uses	An anodyne for relief of pain. Also as a demulcent for soothing coughs and colds. Can also be used to reduce piles.
Prepared as	Infusion.

Houseleek
SEMPERVIVUM TECTORUM

Found wild	Throughout Britain.
Appearance	A small procumbent plant.
Part used	Leaves.
Therapeutic uses	As an astringent and poultice. Commonly used to soften corns and hard skin.
Prepared as	Infusion and poultice.

Part used	Leaves.
Therapeutic uses	As an astringent and poultice. Commonly used to soften corns and hard skin.
Prepared as	Infusion or poultice.

Hyssop
HYSSOPUS OFFICINALIS

Found wild	UK
Appearance	Small common field herb.
Part used	Leaves.
Therapeutic uses	Stimulant and carminative for bronchial and nasal catarrh. Also for anxiety states and tension.
Prepared as	Infusion.

Iceland Moss
CETRARIA ISLANDICA

Found wild	Throughout Northern Hemisphere.
Appearance	This is not a moss but a procumbent grey lichen.
Part used	Plant.
Therapeutic uses	For catarrh and bronchitis. It is a nutritive and helpful for digestive disorders in small doses.
Prepared as	Decoction.

Irish Moss
CHONDRUS CRISPUS

Also known as	Carragheen Moss.
Found wild	European and North American coasts.
Appearance	Small, procumbent seaweed with fan-shaped fronds.
Part used	Whole plant.
Therapeutic uses	Mainly in cough medicines for its demulcent properties. It is nutritious and can be used as a food. Externally as a lotion for dermatitis and roughened hands.
Prepared as	Infusion.

Jaborandi
PILOCARPUS MICROPHYLLUS

Found wild	Brazil.
Appearance	A small herb.
Part used	Leaves.
Therapeutic uses	A diaphoretic and expectorant. Also beneficial to asthma sufferers.
Prepared as	Decoction — external use only. Restricted purchase only. Usually sold as one part Jaborandi to 19 parts Rosemary.

Kava
PIPER METHYSTICUM

Also known as	Kava-Kava.
Found wild	South Pacific.
Appearance	Tall shrub.
Part used	Root.
Therapeutic uses	As a tonic and a diuretic. Helpful for the treatment of joint pains, rheumatism and gout.
Prepared as	Decoction.

Kola
COLA VERA

Also known as	Kola Nut and Cola Nut.
Found wild	West Africa.
Appearance	A large tree of outstanding elegance.
Part used	Seeds.
Therapeutic uses	Nerve stimulant and heart tonic.
Prepared as	Powder.

Lady's Slipper
CYPRIPEDIUM PRUBESCENS

Also known as	Nerveroot.
Found wild	Europe and USA.
Appearance	A delicate white orchid.
Part used	Rhizome.

Therapeutic uses	An effective nervine, valuable in cases of tension and anxiety. Tonic. Sedative.
Prepared as	Infusion.

Lavender
LAVANDULA OFFICINALIS

Found wild	UK and Europe.
Appearance	Familiar garden plant with grey needle-like leaves.
Part used	Flowers.
Therapeutic uses	Carminative and stimulant. Used for depressive headaches.
Prepared as	Infusion and oil.

Lettuce, Wild
LACTUCA VIROSA

Found wild	Warm parts of Europe.
Appearance	A small plant of bushy appearance.
Parts used	Leaves and juice.
Therapeutic uses	An anodyne and sedative. Also useful to ease coughs of nervous origin. Relieves rheumatic pain.
Prepared as	Decoction.

Linseed
LINUM USITATISSIMUM

Also known as	Flax Seed.
Found wild	Worldwide.
Appearance	An erect plant with strong fleshy leaves.
Part used	Seed.
Therapeutic uses	Pectoral demulcent and emollient. As a poultice for boils and carbuncles.
Prepared as	Infusion or poultice.

Liquorice
GLYCYRRHIZA GLABRA

Found wild	Europe and Middle East.
Appearance	A strong-growing perennial plant.
Part used	Root.
Therapeutic uses	In cough medicines. As a demulcent and pectoral and as a gentle laxative.
Prepared as	Decoction.

Logwood
HAEMATOXYLON CAMPECHIANUM

Found wild	South America.
Appearance	A massive tree.
Part used	Wood.

| **Therapeutic uses** | To relieve diarrhoea and dysentery. Also helpful for slight haemorrhaging from uterus. |
| **Prepared as** | Decoction. |

Manna
FRAXINUS ORNUS

Found wild	Mediterranean countries.
Appearance	Medium-sized shrub.
Part used	Sap from cuts in bark.
Therapeutic uses	As a gentle laxative for pregnant women, and as a nutritive invalid food.
Prepared as	Decoction.

Marigold
CALENDULA OFFICINALIS

Found wild	Throughout northern hemisphere.
Appearance	Small plant with attractive yellow flowers.
Parts used	Petals and leaves.
Therapeutic uses	A stimulant, diaphoretic and anti-inflammatory. External application helps varicose veins and skin ulcers. A general antiseptic.
Prepared as	Infusion or ointment.

Therapeutic uses	An antispasmodic with marked tonic qualities. Excellent for migraine.
Prepared as	Infusion.

Meadowsweet
FILIPENDULA ULMARIA

Also known as	Bridewort.
Found wild	UK and Europe.
Appearance	Long-stemmed herb growing almost one metre.
Part used	Herb.
Therapeutic uses	Anti-rheumatic, stomachic, astringent. Helpful for severe cases of cystitis. Muscular, rheumatic and joint pains.
Prepared as	Infusion.

Motherwort
LEONURUS CARDIACA

Where found	A common garden plant in Britain and northern Europe.
Appearance	A pink-flowered shrub.
Part used	Herb.
Therapeutic uses	A nervine and for the relief of menopausal symptoms. Also a tonic and stimulant and helpful for heart conditions.
Prepared as	Infusion.

Mullein
VERBASCUM THAPSUS

Found wild	Throughout Europe.
Appearance	Tall perennial cylindrical plant with a tower of yellow flowers.
Part used	Leaves and flowers.
Therapeutic uses	For lung and bronchial inflammations. As an astringent, demulcent and pectoral.
Prepared as	Infusion.

Night Blooming Cereus
CEREUS GRANDIFLORUS

Found wild	Jamaica.
Appearance	A small branded cactus with large creamy flowers.
Part used	Plant.
Therapeutic uses	An effective heart stimulant and for relief of palpitations. Also a diuretic and helpful for prostate diseases.
Prepared as	Decoction.

Nutmeg
MYRISTICA FRAGRANS

Found wild	Malaysia, Indonesia and the West Indies.
Appearance	Tall tree.
Part used	Seeds and oil.

Appearance	A pink-flowered shrub of handsome appearance.
Part used	Herb.
Therapeutic uses	A nervine and for the relief of amenorrhea in women. Also a tonic and stimulant. It is helpful for heart conditions.
Prepared as	Infusion.

Mountain Grape
BERBERIS AQUIFOLIUM

Also known as	Oregon Grape.
Found wild	USA and Canada.
Appearance	Tall-growing plant with small yellow flowers.
Part used	Root.
Therapeutic uses	Tonic, mild laxative and alterative. Of great help in skin conditions such as psoriasis and eczema.
Prepared as	Decoction.

Mullein
VERBASCUM THAPSUS

Found wild	Throughout Europe.
Appearance	Tall, perennial, cylindrical plant with a tower of yellow flowers.
Parts used	Leaves and flowers.

Therapeutic uses	For lung and bronchial inflammations. As an astringent, demulcent and pectoral.
Prepared as	Infusion.

Night Blooming Cereus
CEREUS GRANDIFLORUS

Found wild	Jamaica.
Appearance	Small branded cactus with large creamy flowers.
Part used	Plant.
Therapeutic uses	An effective heart stimulant which also relieves palpitations. Also a diuretic and helpful for prostate diseases.
Prepared as	Decoction.

Nutmeg
MYRISTICA FRAGRANS

Found wild	Malaysia, Indonesia and the West Indies.
Appearance	Tall tree.
Part used	Seeds and oil.
Therapeutic uses	Carminative and anti-emetic. Helpful in most cases of stomach upset. Can be used externally for the treatment of rheumatic pain. Use in moderation.
Prepared as	Powder or oil.

Appearance	A low-growing herb with tiny green flowers. Not related to common parsley.
Part used	Herb.
Therapeutic uses	For the relief of bladder and kidney troubles and helpful in dissolving kidney stones.
Prepared as	Infusion.

Parsley Root
PETROSELINUM CRISPUM

Found wild	UK and Europe.
Appearance	Small herb.
Part used	Root.
Therapeutic uses	Carminative, diuretic, emmenagogue. Has useful anti-rheumatic properties.
Prepared as	Decoction.

Passion Flower
PASSIFLORA INCARNATA

Also known as	Maypop.
Found wild	Worldwide in warm climates.
Appearance	Climbing plant with purple fruits.
Parts used	Stem and leaves.
Therapeutic uses	Sedative, narcotic, antispasmodic. useful for insomnia.
Prepared as	Infusion.

Pennyroyal
MENTHA PULEGIUM

Found wild	UK and Europe.
Appearance	Low-growing herb.
Parts used	Herb and oil.
Therapeutic uses	Carminative, emmenagogue, stimulant, diaphoretic. This herb has always been regarded as reliable treatment for obstructed menstruation. Contraindicated in pregnancy. Applied externally it is helpful for gout.
Prepared as	Infusion.

Peony
PAEONIA OFFICINALIS

Found wild	Southern Asia.
Appearance	Beautiful perennial that bears vivid double flowers in profusion.
Part used	Root.
Therapeutic uses	Antispasmodic and tonic.
Prepared as	Infusion.

Peppermint
MENTHA PIPERITA

Also known as	Curled Mint.
Found wild	Europe and North America.
Appearance	A stately herb with purple-hued stems.

Prepared as   Infusion.

Parsley Root
PETROSELINUM CRISPUM

Found wild	UK and Europe.
Appearance	Small herb.
Part used	Root.
Therapeutic uses	Carminative, diuretic, and an emmenagogue. Has useful anti-rheumatic properties.
Prepared as	Decoction.

Pennyroyal
MENTHA PULEGIUM

Found wild	UK and Europe.
Appearance	Low-growing herb.
Parts used	Herb and oil.
Therapeutic uses	Carminative, emmenagogue, stimulant and diaphoretic. This herb has always been regarded as reliable treatment for obstructed menstruation. Applied externally it is helpful for gout.
Prepared as	Infusion. Contraindicated in pregnancy.

Peony
PAEONIA OFFICINALIS

Found wild	Southern Asia.
Appearance	Beautiful perennial that bears vivid double flowers in profusion.
Part used	Root.
Therapeutic uses	Antispasmodic and tonic.
Prepared as	Infusion.

Peppermint
MENTHA PIPERITA

Also known as	Curled Mint.
Found wild	Europe and North America.
Appearance	A stately herb with purple-hued stems and pink flowers.
Part used	Herb.
Therapeutic uses	A stomachic and carminative. Also relieves sickness, flatulence and indigestion.
Prepared as	Infusion.

Periwinkle (South African)
VINCA ROSA

Found wild	South Africa.
Appearance	Large, trailing herb with profuse pink flowers.
Part used	Herb.
Therapeutic uses	Helpful for treatment of diabetes.
Prepared as	Infusion.

| Therapeutic uses | Diaphoretic, carminative, stimulant. Helpful for circulation disorders associated with rheumatism. |
| Prepared as | Decoction. |

Pulsatilla
ANEMONE PULSATILLA

Also known as	Wind Flower.
Found wild	UK and Europe.
Appearance	A large weed with purple flowers.
Part used	Leaves.
Therapeutic uses	Sedative, nervine, antispasmodic. Helpful for women with menstrual problems and also for headaches associated with tension. Insomnia. Skin eruptions.
Prepared as	Infusion.

Quassia
PICRAENA EXCELSA

Found wild	West Indies.
Appearance	A tree of great stature.
Part used	Wood.
Therapeutic uses	As a tonic and also effective for treatment of stomach disorders. Helpful for cramp.
Prepared as	Infusion.

Raspberry
RUBUS IDAEUS

Where found	Commonly cultivated in most temperate climates.
Appearance	A bush producing edible fruit.
Part used	Leaves.
Therapeutic uses	Astringent and stimulant. Useful in the treatment of painful periods, easier childbirth, and also as a gargle for sore throat.
Prepared as	Infusion.

Red Sage
SALVIA OFFICINALIS

Also known as	Sage.
Found wild	Europe and North America.
Appearance	A small herb.
Part used	Leaves.
Therapeutic uses	An astringent, helpful for sore throats, quinsy and laryngitis.
Prepared as	Infusion.

Rosemary
ROSMARINUS OFFICINALIS

Found wild	UK and Europe.
Appearance	Evergreen shrub with fragrant needle-type leaves.
Part used	Leaves.

Queen's Delight
STILLINGIA SYLVATICA

Found wild	United States.
Appearance	A perrenial herb.
Part used	Root.
Therapeutic uses	A blood purifier used in mixtures for skin diseases. Also a laxative and diuretic.
Prepared as	Powder, decoction.

Raspberry
RUBUS IDAEUS

Where found	Commonly cultivated in most temperate climates.
Appearance	A bush producing edible fruit.
Part used	Leaves.
Therapeutic uses	Astringent and stimulant. Useful in the treatment of painful periods, easier childbirth, and also as a gargle for sore throat.
Prepared as	Infusion.

Red Clover
TRIFOLIUM PRATENSE

Also known as	Trefoil.
Found wild	Europe.
Appearance	A common clover.
Part used	Whole.

Therapeutic uses	A sedative and alterative. Used externally for psoriasis and eczema.
Prepared as	Infusion.

Red Sage
SALVIA OFFICINALIS

Also known as	Sage.
Found wild	Europe and North America.
Appearance	A small herb.
Part used	Leaves.
Therapeutic uses	An astringent, helpful for sore throats, quinsy and laryngitis.
Prepared as	Infusion.

St John's Wort
HYPERICUM PERFORATUM

Found wild	Great Britain.
Appearance	Sturdy yellow-flowered herb.
Part used	Herb.
Therapeutic uses	Diuretic and expectorant, helpful for coughs and bronchial ailments.
Prepared as	Decoction.

Samphire
CRITHMUM MARITIMUM

Also known as	Rock Samphire.

| **Therapeutic uses** | Famous as a nervine and tonic, it relieves nervous tension and tremor. Scullcap is prescribed for a wide range of nervous disorders. |
| **Prepared as** | Infusion. |

Senna
CASSIA AUGUSTIFOLIA

Found wild	Arabia.
Appearance	Tree of sparse growth with distinctive grey-green leaves.
Parts used	Leaves and seed case.
Therapeutic uses	A safe laxative without purging effect. Combine with ginger.
Prepared as	Infusion.

Shepherd's Purse
CAPSELLA BURSA-PASTORIS

Found wild	Everywhere.
Appearance	Small insignificant weed with little white flowers.
Part used	Herb.
Therapeutic uses	Diuretic, usually for kidney and urinary troubles. Antiscorbutic.
Prepared as	Infusion.

Slippery Elm
ULMUS FULVA

Found wild	North America.
Appearance	A great tree of spreading growth.
Part used	Inner part of bark.
Therapeutic uses	As a nutritive for invalids. Also an emollient and demulcent for healing burns and skin troubles.
Prepared as	Infusion and powder.

Spearmint
MENTHA VIRIDIS

Found wild	Throughout the northern hemisphere.
Appearance	Strong-growing perennial herb.
Therapeutic uses	Stimulant. Carminative. Suitable for the very young and old.
Prepared as	Infusion.

Squaw Weed
SENECIO AUREUS

Also known as	Life Root Plant and Golden Senecio.
Found wild	UK, Europe and the United States.
Appearance	Common herb.
Parts used	Rhizome and leaves.
Therapeutic uses	Diuretic. Astringent. Tonic. Menopausal neurosis.
Prepared as	Infusion.

| **Prepared as** | Infusion and powder. |

Spearmint
MENTHA VIRIDIS

Found wild	Throughout the northern hemisphere.
Appearance	Strong-growing perennial herb.
Therapeutic uses	A stimulant and carminative, suitable for the very young and old.
Prepared as	Infusion.

Squill
URFINEA MARITIMA

Found wild	Southern Europe and North Africa.
Appearance	One of the lily family.
Part used	Corm.
Therapeutic uses	Expectorant, helpful in relieving catarrh, asthma and bronchial troubles. Also a cathartic and diuretic.
Prepared as	Decoction.

Swamp Milkweed
ASCLEPIAS INCARNATA

| **Found wild** | United States. |
| **Appearance** | Medium-size shrub of grotesque appearance. |

Parts used	Rhizome and root.
Therapeutic uses	A cathartic and an emetic, beneficial in the treatment of arthritis and stomach disorders.
Prepared as	Infusion. Small doses.

Sweet Chestnut
CASTANEA SATIVA

Found wild	UK and Europe.
Appearance	Large tree.
Part used	Leaves.
Therapeutic uses	Astringent and anti-rheumatic. Helpful in cases of muscular rheumatism, lumbago and fibrositis and of specific benefit to catarrhal conditions.
Prepared as	Infusion.

Sweet Sumach
RHUS AROMATICA

Where found	Canada and the United States.
Appearance	A shrub growing to about 4ft high.
Part used	Root-bark.
Therapeutic uses	Astringent and diuretic used in the treatment of incontinence in children and in the elderly.
Prepared as	Infusion.

Thyme
THYMUS VULGARIS

Where found	Common garden plant.
Appearance	Small perennial herb with tiny leaves.
Part used	Herb.
Therapeutic uses	Antispasmodic and tonic. Contains thymol, a strong antiseptic, useful in irritable coughs and catarrh.
Prepared as	Infusion is sweetened with honey and given in tablespoonful doses.

Valerian
VALERIANA OFFICINALIS

Found wild	UK.
Appearance	A small herb.
Part used	Rhizome.
Therapeutic uses	Anodyne, sedative, nervine. Excellent for relieving nervous tension or nervous debility. Promotes sleep.
Prepared as	Decoction.

Vervain
VERBENA OFFICINALIS

Found wild	UK.
Appearance	Small trailing herb.
Part used	Leaves.
Therapeutic uses	Tonic. Sudorific. Emetic. A very good nervine to help depression and tension.
Prepared as	Infusion.

Water Dock
RUMEX AQUATICUS

Also known as	Bloodwort.
Found wild	Throughout Europe.
Appearance	One of the common dock family.
Part used	Root.
Therapeutic uses	An alterative and detergent. Helps clean and strengthen gums and relieves mouth ulcers.
Prepared as	Infusion.

Wild Carrot
CAUCUS CAROTA

Found wild	UK and Europe.
Appearance	Small version of cultivated carrot.
Part used	Herb.
Therapeutic uses	Diuretic, carminative. Helpful in cases of cystitis, bladder infection and gout.
Prepared as	Infusion.

Prepared as   Decoction.

Wild Carrot
DAUCUS CAROTA

Found wild	UK and Europe.
Appearance	Small version of cultivated carrot.
Part used	Herb.
Therapeutic uses	A diuretic, carminative. Helpful in cases of cystitis, bladder infection and gout.
Prepared as	Infusion.

Wild Indigo
BAPTISIA TINCTORIA

Also known as	Indigo Weed.
Found wild	USA and Canada.
Appearance	Medium-sized shrub.
Parts used	Root and leaves.
Therapeutic uses	An antiseptic and stimulant. Used externally for ulcers and boils.
Prepared as	Infusion or ointment.

Wild Yam Root
DIOSCOREA VILLOSA

Also known as	Rheumatism Root. Colic Root.
Found wild	North America and tropical areas.
Appearance	Tuberous plant.
Part used	Root.

Therapeutic uses	An anti-inflammatory, antispasmodic and diaphoretic. Helpful in the treatment of rheumatoid arthritis and muscular rheumatism. Leg cramps and intermittent claudication are two other conditions which can be beneficially treated.
Prepared as	Decoction.

Wood Sage
TEUCRIUM SCORODONIA

Also known as	Garlic Sage.
Found wild	UK.
Appearance	Herb.
Part used	Herb.
Therapeutic uses	For respiratory infections. An astringent and anti-rheumatic. This herb has been used for many years to treat respiratory infections, rheumatic pain and stiffness.
Prepared as	Infusion.

Yarrow
ACHILLEA MILLEFOLIUM

Also known as	Milfoil.
Found wild	Great Britain.
Appearance	A tiny herb.

A guide to herbal suppliers

Medical herbalists practise in most towns, while health food shops should be able to assist with the more common dried herbs. Specialist requirements, though, often need specialist stockists.

The following list is by no means complete, but should be sufficient to cover most herbs mentioned in this book.

MAIL ORDER STOCKISTS

Cathay of Bournemouth Ltd
3 Wickham Road
Bournemouth
Dorset
BH7 6JX
(Free literature on request.)

Culpeper Ltd
Hadstock Road
Linton
Cambs
CB1 6NJ

MAJOR RETAIL OUTLETS

Bournemouth   Cathay of Bournemouth Ltd
3 Wickham Road
Bournemouth
Dorset
BH7 6JX

Gerard House
736 Christchurch Road
Bournemouth,
and

	31 St Thomas Street
	Lymington
	Hants
Edinburgh	Napiers of Edinburgh
	18 Bristo Place
	Edinburgh
	EH1 1EZ
London	G. Baldwin
	173 Walworth Road
	London
	SE17 1RW
	Neal's Yard Remedies
	Neal's Yard
	Covent Garden
	London
	WC2H 9DP
Ryde	The Grail
	1 The High Street
	Ryde
	Isle of Wight
	PO33 2PN

Culpeper Herbal Shops can be found in nine major towns, including three in London.

A directory of medical herbalists is available from the National Institute of Medical Herbalists, 9 Palace Gate, Exeter, Devon, EX1 1JA. It is advisable to consult a medical herbalist if any doubt still exists about a particular condition or suggested remedy.

Glossary of common medical terms

Very often when reading, or on having a medical consultation, words are used which may not be familiar. This short list will help to make some of the more common ones a little clearer.

Alterative   Any substance that can beneficially alter the condition of a patient.

Amenorrhoea   Cessation of the menstrual flow.

Anodyne   Any substance which eases pain.

Antiseptic   Any substance that prevents putrefaction.

Antispasmodic   Any substance that prevents or relieves spasms.

Anthelmintic   Any herb acting against intestinal worms.

Aperient   Any substance producing the natural evacuation of the bowels.

Aphrodisiac   Any substance that stimulates sexual functions.

Astringent	Any substance which causes contraction of body tissues.
Cardiac	Any condition affecting or pertaining to the heart.
Carminative	Any substance that relieves pain caused by flatulence.
Cathartic	Any substance that induces stimulation of bowel action; rather stronger than aperients.
Corrective	Any substance that restores normal conditions.
Debility	Feebleness of health.
Degenerative	Deterioration or change in tissue structure.
Demulcent	Any soothing medicine.
Deobstruent	Any substance that frees the natural orifices of the body.
Diaphoretic	Any substance inducing perspiration.
Diuretic	Any substance that increases the flow of urine.
Dysmenorrhoea	Excessive pain during menstruation.

Emetic

Any substance that causes vomiting.

Emmenagogue

Any drug that stimulates menstruation.

Emollient

Any substance that soothes and lubricates.

Haemostatic

Any substance that checks bleeding and aids the clotting of blood.

Insecticide

Any substance that is fatal to insects.

Laxative

Any substance that induces gentle, easy bowel action.

Leucorrhea

Any mucus discharge from female genitals.

Menorrhagia

Excessive flow in menstruation.

Myalgia

Any muscular rheumatic pain.

Narcotic

Any drug that induces stupor and insensibility.

Nephritic

Any drug that affects the kidneys.

Nervine

Any substance that restores the nerves to a normal tone.

Oxytocic

Any drug that contracts the uterus and hastens childbirth.

Parturient   Any product used during childbirth.

Resolvent   Any substance that reduces swelling.

Rubefacient   Any substance that produces inflammation of the skin.

Sedative   Any substance used to placate 'nerves'.

Soporific   Any substance used to promote sleep.

Stimulant   Any substance used to promote the reserve power of the body and produce strength and energy.

Stomachic   Any substance that allays stomach disorders.

Styptic   Any substance that aids the clotting of blood.

Sudorific   Any substance producing heavy perspiration.

Tonic   Any substance that, if used regularly, will promote vivacity and well being.

Vermifuge   Any substance that expels worms from the body.

Vulnerary   Any substance that promotes the healing of wounds.

FURTHER READING

Other books in this Herbal Series include:

Stress and Tension
Arthritis and Rheumatism
Sexual Problems

Other Foulsham books on herbal medicine edited by David Potterton include:

Culpeper's Colour Herbal
Medicinal Plants